I'M GLAD I GOT CANCER

A SURVIVOR'S GUIDE TO OVERCOMING ADVERSITY

KELLY WILTON

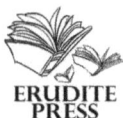

ERUDITE
PRESS

ISBN: 978-1-937979-95-9

Erudite Press

Goshen, Kentucky 40026

www.eruditepress.com

DEDICATION

I would like to posthumously acknowledge my Dad, for unwittingly providing the inspiration for this book.

In loving memory of my Mom, who chose a different path in her cancer battle, which opened my eyes to the power of choice.

I also wish to honor Rita, who has inspired me in so many ways — during my fight with cancer, during her fight with cancer, and during the cancer-free years that have followed for both of us.

And finally, I would like to thank the staff of University of Michigan Comprehensive Cancer Center.

PREFACE

When faced with an unplanned and unwanted obstacle in life, what do you do? Some may give up and let the obstacle define the rest of their lives. They may turn to drugs, alcohol, or other substances to dull the pain. They may become bitter and complain to all who will listen about how unfair life is. Some may stay stuck in their new reality, not actively destroying themselves, but not fully living either. Others may dig deep and find the strength, courage, and perseverance to overcome the obstacle, and come out the other side a much stronger, better, and more resilient version of themselves. So who chooses your outcome? You do! When faced with a life-altering moment, the paths to choose from are limitless. This is the time to decide if the one you chose is serving you well. And if not, you may choose another.

This book is my very personal account of overcoming cancer. I was diagnosed with Stage III rectal cancer at the age of forty-six. After fourteen months of battling with the disease, and several more months recovering from the treatment, all tests and scans show that I remain cancer-free. I now count myself as a six-year cancer survivor. Many of my friends told me how easy I made it all seem— they said I never appeared "sick" physically, mentally, or emotionally, and went about fighting for my life with barely a ripple. Throughout the process, I knew I wanted to tell my story so that others could learn from my experience, but I couldn't really envision what form it would take. And then it came to me.

About midway through my ordeal, my father who has since passed away, made a comment that became the catalyst for this book; but first, a little background on him. At seventy-two years old, dad's health was not great: he had congestive heart failure, kidney disease, a kidney transplant, a heart attack, at least one major and several minor strokes, was nearly blind from glaucoma, and could walk for no more than five minutes before his hip started hurting too much. We were sitting in his living room, chatting about nothing in particular, with the TV on in the background, when out of the blue he said, "Kelly, I'm glad you got cancer."

My first thought was, *Dad's had another stroke.* My

second thought was, *Was there a mix-up with his medications?* But then he went on to say, "I'm not **glad** you got cancer, I'm glad **you** got cancer instead of one of your sisters." This clarification didn't make things much better, but I thought I should let him say what was on his mind.

He continued, "You have a great job that is giving you the flexibility you need, you have good insurance coverage, and you have some money in the bank. So from a financial and career standpoint, you are going to be okay. But, more than that, you have the right attitude. I don't know how to describe it, but your attitude makes you able to cope with everything just fine. I don't think your sisters have that. They are more like your mother, and you are more like me." My mother died from cancer at age sixty-two, and from the minute she was diagnosed, she felt helpless, hopeless, and easily overwhelmed. She lost all sense of perspective. She couldn't distinguish between a minor issue and a major challenge; everything became an enormous obstacle that she had to struggle with, and always felt like she came up short.

So after a few hugs between Dad and me, a few tears all around, and me assuring Dad that each of my sisters would surprise him with their fighting attitude if cornered by an adversary such as cancer, I began to try to dissect what, specifically, went into this "attitude" he was talking about, and the ease which my friends claimed I exhibited.

I don't think I changed overnight when I was diagnosed with cancer. This attitude was in me all along, and cancer just gave me the stage to showcase it. If I wanted to do a proper job of deconstructing the winning attitude, I knew I would need to dig deep. I would need to go way back through key life experiences to explore the events, actions, and beliefs that prepared me to overcome this huge battle. And that, my friends, is how this book was born. I invite you to journey with me.

———

Before we get started, however, I need to tell you that you will read nothing new here. I don't claim to have found The Answer. All of the ideas and concepts I share are drawn from information I have gathered through reading books on a wide variety of topics, including psychology, spirituality, business management, even diet and fitness, and from having fascinating conversations with people who are always striving for greater knowledge and personal insight. I include information that resonates with me, that describes my experience, and just seems "right." My experience is just that: my unique experience.

There are more than 200 different types of

cancer, each with dozens of possible symptoms. Each type of cancer has a multitude of different treatment options, each with its own set of potential side effects. The math, alone, says that out of a million patients with cancer, there can be a million different experiences. It would be impractical to assume that anyone reading this book will have the exact same experiences I did. Hopefully, you will be able to connect with at least some of my experience and utilize some of the lessons I have learned.

Although most of the examples and stories I use throughout this book reference my specific battle with cancer, I hope the deeper information and insight resonate with you, and the underlying message in each chapter may be utilized, regardless of what difficult situation you are facing in your life.

1

WHERE IS YOUR FOCUS?

During the summer of 2012, I was living and working in London, England. I had been there just over one year, working as a Customs & Freight Manager for a global supply chain company sponsoring the London 2012 Olympic Games. This was a very high-profile assignment; I was in charge of importing all of the items needed to stage the Games, working closely with the organizing committee, global broadcast and press agencies, and the Olympic committees from each participating nation. This was the opportunity of a lifetime, and I was enjoying every minute of it. Imagine me, raised in a run-down farmhouse in the outskirts of a small town in the middle of nowhere, not only living in one of the largest and most dynamic cities in the world, but working with colleagues who were world travelers—

people who had made the Olympics their career by following the Games from host city to host city.

On the job, the level of excitement and sense of purpose was heady. We were all performing at our best, knowing that failure was not an option. I had spent the past year in preparation and had recently hired a team that would support me throughout the Games. My team consisted of people from the USA, Australia, France, Italy, Czech Republic and, of course, England. I was trying to compress my thirty years of import/export knowledge and experience into two weeks of intensive training for a group of people who not only had no relevant experience, but most could barely understand my American English. We were all working twelve to fourteen hours a day, but it didn't seem to matter since "work" had begun to take on a carnival atmosphere over the past several months.

I had been experiencing fatigue and physical discomfort for months (to avoid being unnecessarily graphic, I'll just say I was having bathroom issues). I self-diagnosed it as something that would go away on its own, like hemorrhoids. I did not see a doctor for confirmation, primarily because I was too busy with work, but also because it never occurred to me that it might be something serious. The closer the big day got, the longer my work hours became. And unfortunately, the pain and exhaustion became unbearable.

In early July, I finally saw a doctor and had the rug pulled out from under my feet. I will always remember the look of compassion on the doctor's face and his first words after he completed the examination: "I'm sorry, you have cancer."

"Devastated" does not begin to describe how I felt. But immediately, I knew I had to make my first choice: I could either allow feelings of unfairness to derail and distract me, or I could focus on the task at hand and confront the next steps head-on. It was easy in the beginning, since I knew time was of the essence on the job. I had to assist my manager with quickly finding a replacement for me because we knew my team was not ready to operate during Games-time without a strong leader.

I had to give up my apartment, pack my belongings, close my bank account, and do all of the other things a person needs to do to wrap up an overseas assignment and leave the country. These details kept me busy enough that I had no time for worry and regret.

Once I returned home, however, it became more difficult to keep my focus away from "what should have been" if I had stayed on my assignment. There were a lot of things I was looking forward to and I felt regret for missing the "fun part" of the job. For example, I returned home just days before the Opening Ceremony. I also had tickets to the final dress rehearsal of the Opening Ceremony, tickets to several competition events, and had all-access passes to some of the venues. I felt I was being ripped away from the excitement of the Games, making the feelings of loss even more dreadful.

I was also disappointed that I would be unable to finish my assignment and would not having the opportunity to enjoy the fruits of my labor at the conclusion of the project. It was unfair that I didn't return home the "conquering hero" and bask in the glory of having successfully completed the high-profile work assignment that was supposed to have catapulted my career into the stratosphere.

Instead, what actually happened was that I came home quietly. Out of respect for my privacy, no mention was made to my work colleagues about the circumstances of my return. I was given a new, low-stress assignment which would allow me to work from home while undergoing treatment. I worried about the direction my career would take once I became cancer-free, but I knew for certain that it was no longer on the same trajectory as before.

I had moments of anger because of the unfairness of it all: anger at fate, anger at the cancer, anger at God, and anger at myself for not seeing a doctor as soon as the symptoms first appeared. The cancer was causing my professional life to take an unexpected, and unwanted, turn. It was causing untold physical pain and discomfort that I knew would only get worse. And I worried that all of the scars, both physical and emotional, were going to negatively impact my intimate relationships. However, I could not allow these feelings to interfere with my healing. I knew that staying stuck in "should-have-been" and "if only" did not serve my purpose.

Instead of looking backwards, I focused entirely on "what happens next?" I started each day with the thought, *What do I need to do today to not only survive, but thrive?* Then I just did it — one day at a time, with no drama, and no fuss. I also made it my business to ask questions about what to expect every step of the way. By keeping my focus on current actions and the next steps, I was able to recognize and celebrate small milestones. I had a clear vision of my end goal: cancer-free and healthy. Every action I took was in support of that goal.

2

WHAT STORY ARE YOU TELLING YOURSELF?

A huge component of being successful is not allowing past failures, or old stories and limitations, to stand in your way. Many years ago, I did some personal growth work where we learned how, as small children, we come to believe certain things about ourselves. These beliefs can show up in the most annoying ways as adults, and they can unknowingly stop us from achieving what we want.

For example, my bottom-line, underlying limiting belief about myself has always been: "I'm not good enough." I quickly realized that, if I had gone into battle with that story from my past running in the background, I would not be successful: I would be "not be good enough" to withstand the side effects of treatment; the chemo/radiation would be "not be good enough" to shrink the tumor; the surgeons would be "not be good enough" to remove all of the cancer; my care-givers would be "not be good enough" to deal with wound healing, and so on.

Instead, I recognized this bottom-line negative belief, and acknowledged that it would not serve me well. So I continuously brought to mind my highest vision of my highest self: **"I am able."** Therefore, by extension, everyone and everything that was in support of my goal was also "able"—I created the experience of everyone around me being "able": my radiologist was "able" to shrink the tumor; my surgeon was "able" to remove all of the cancer; my friends and family were "able" to support me in exactly the right ways.

Can you imagine living in a world where you know, I mean *really know*, that everyone around you is "able?" It really was life-changing for me to be able to hold myself, and others, in the space of "able," fully trusting in our combined abilities to bring me through. This left little room for worry, or fear.

In the past, I had seen others as "able" only sporadically. I have one friend who said to me a few years ago, "Kelly, you have always seen me as being bigger than I see myself. I am proud to say that I have finally grown into the person you always knew I was." Even knowing what an impact my belief in this friend had on how he saw himself, I was quite stingy and selective in seeing others as able. It was only after seeing, firsthand, the very real benefits of projecting "able" onto others that I became more intentional about seeing everyone I interact with as "able"... and they generally deliver!

During the personal growth work mentioned earlier, I learned that your bottom-line limiting beliefs can take many forms. Some examples are:

- I am not enough
- I am not important
- I am stupid
- I am unlovable
- I am a failure
- I am damaged

I found it very helpful to go through the exercise of determining what my bottom-line, limiting belief was—just to "connect the dots" on why my life has played out the way it has.

1. To help determine what your limiting beliefs are, first find a quiet place and clear your mind. When you are relaxed, **think back to your earliest negative memory.** By negative, I mean sad, lonely, scared, angry, hurt, etc. The earliest

memory I identified was from the first grade. I had made a new friend, and she and I were on the playground during recess. It was cold outside, so I asked her to wait for me while I went inside to get my mittens. When I returned, she was gone. In retrospect, I can think of a dozen reasons she may have not waited around for me — maybe I wasn't clear that I would return quickly, maybe she got cold and wanted to run around on the playground, maybe she had to use the bathroom, maybe, maybe, maybe. Regardless of the reason she left, in the moment, I was devastated. You may be thinking that this is a silly little event that should not have had any impact on my life. As a child, however, sometimes the most innocuous thing can have a tremendous impact; don't judge the memory that comes to mind for you...it could be something big and heartbreaking (such as abuse, abandonment, or betrayal) or it could be something that seems silly and inconsequential, like mine. This event, and the meaning your younger self attached to it, can have significant impact on the rest of your life—if you allow it.

The next step is to **ask yourself how that experience made you feel.** Then open yourself up to that feeling — really experience it again. Immerse yourself in those feelings. In my childhood story, I was lonely and hurt. Once you are fully experiencing your feelings, ask yourself, "What did that experience mean about me?" You may need to work with this a bit. Our first natural response is generally about the other person. In my experience in the first grade, my initial thoughts were: *She didn't think I was important enough*, and *She just didn't care about me*. Keep working until you get clarity on what story you made up at the time to tell yourself what the event meant about you. You need to get past what the event meant **to** you and arrive at what it meant **about** you. For me, it was: *I'm not good enough*.

During this exercise, as soon as that thought occurred to me, it resonated through my whole body, and I started shaking because of how true it felt. It instantly became clear how I had let that belief define me throughout life. For one, I have struggled with finding a life partner; the persistent belief was: *I'm not good enough to attract and keep a nice man*. Because of this belief, I have never held a long-term, committed relationship. For another, I generally manage to get "this close" to my goals then fall apart. I managed to lose seventy pounds once and wanted to lose another twenty-five pounds. Things were going smoothly until *I'm not good enough to finish this* got in the way, and I regained forty pounds. I could go on for pages with examples of how the subconscious belief of *I'm not good enough* has influenced my decision-making. But I don't want to spend any more time, or attention, on the past than is needed to make my point. So we will move onward.

Please know that the stories that you told yourself as a child are not "The Truth." They are just stories you made up to explain what happened, and you decided to believe them. So, now that you remember what the stories are that have been limiting your success, what do you do? It's easy: you **make up new stories.** You change the narrative.

Recognize and acknowledge when a limiting belief is running things. At first, it will be something like, *Oh, it was six-year-old Kelly's story of 'not good enough' that stopped me from starting a conversation with that nice-looking man a few hours ago.* Eventually, you will be able to spot your bottom-line belief when you are in the middle of it, thus allowing you to consciously adopt a new belief. This is where you get to **define your highest vision of your highest self.**

For me, the opposite of *I'm not good enough* looks like is *I am able.* When you are at your best—clicking on all cylinders, so to speak—what do you think about yourself? Maybe for you, the opposite of *I am damaged* is *I am whole.* Whatever words you choose to describe yourself will be right and perfect. The great news is that you get to choose whichever belief serves you best. For example, if you believe that you are unlovable, the laws of attraction will put you in situations that prove just how unlovable you are. But if you believe you are lovable and loving, you will create loving and reciprocal relationships.

My story of *I am able* is what got me to London and the Olympics in the first place. *I'm not good enough* has not shown up at work in years. I started working in my field when I was still in high school, as a general office clerk, earning minimum wage, with no benefits. I made copies, I filed, I stuffed envelopes, I filled in for the receptionist when she was on break, and I did some general data entry. And I learned. I asked questions until I understood the "why" of everything—not just the "what" and the "how." Nearly every day I finished my assigned task with time to spare. So I was always asking my supervisor for more work to do.

After eight years of rotating through nearly every position in the company, and receiving small annual pay increases, I realized that the office in my hometown was too small for me to progress very far. The more senior people were all too young to retire any time soon, and it was unheard of for people to quit or get fired.

I asked the office manager to tell me where he saw me in a few years, and his response was, "Doing the same thing you are doing now." Although I appreciated his frankness, that was not the answer I wanted. So I asked what I needed to do in order to progress in the company.

In the end, I made the huge decision to transfer to our head office in Detroit. Friends, family, and co-workers all thought I was crazy to leave our small town for the big city. Within six months, however, I was promoted to supervisor! My understanding of every aspect of the business—learned over many years of performing nearly every job in my smaller office—helped me to stand head and shoulders above my peers. So, I was the natural choice when a supervisor position became available.

This is the only time that *I'm not good enough* came to the job with me. I really was too young, emotionally and socially, to be a good supervisor. Although I knew the work inside and out, I didn't understand people, and I did not communicate very well. My department yielded good results, but I think it was in spite of me and not because of me. I dealt with self-doubt daily, along with the fear that my inadequacies would be discovered by others.

I had, apparently, become a master at wearing a mask of competency because, within two years, I was promoted again: this time to manager of the department. I now had three supervisors reporting to me. It was during this time that I changed my belief about my work self from *I'm not good enough* to *I am able*. I really grew into the position, and realized that I had a flair for quickly understanding complex concepts and making them understandable to clients and employees alike, and that developing the talents of others was one of my strengths.

For the next twenty years, my career blossomed. I took on new assignments every three to four years — sometimes within the same company, and sometimes accepting positions with new employers — learning something new every time. When I was that naïve seventeen-year old, making copies and filing in Smalltown, USA, I could never have imagined that I would, one day, put the knowledge I was gathering to good use at the Olympics!

For the longest time, I attributed my career success to luck: being in the right place at the right time. But in reality, my belief in my own abilities resulted in performing each job well so that, when opportunities arose, I was the first person the decision-makers thought of. It would never have happened if *I am able* was not continuously running in the background.

Here is a final story for those of you who still don't believe that your personal stories and beliefs create your experience. Growing up, I viewed my family as "poor." In reality, we may not have been "poor" in the truest sense of the word, but my parents certainly did not know how to manage money.

My father earned a decent blue-collar income, but he was supporting a family of six. On at least three occasions, I clearly remember overhearing discussions between my parents about how they needed to make a house payment soon or they would lose the house to foreclosure. These discussions were always followed by visits to my retired grandparents to ask for money. Our electricity and telephone services were shut off for non-payment several times. It took me a long time to figure out why we went to our grandparents' house for dinner every Tuesday night, but I finally connected the dots that Dad's payday was Wednesday, and we had always run out of food and money by Monday or Tuesday. For all of these reasons, and several others too numerous to name here, I grew up with a keen sense of lack. I made a decision at a very early age that *When I'm in charge, I will always have enough money*. I didn't know, or even really care, how I would do that, but I vowed to never live in such financial distress.

For the first twelve years of life as an adult (aged 18-30), I always had enough money. No extra money, but always enough to pay my bills and cover minor emergencies. Because my basic underlying belief was that *I would always have enough*, I subconsciously lived within my means. It was only after I had done the personal growth work discussed earlier, and realized just how powerful our beliefs are, that I decided to get intentional about money.

I changed my story from *I will always have enough money*, to *I have money in abundance*. I still did not know, or care, how it would happen; I just started believing that it would. It was shortly thereafter when I got my first big promotion at work which came with a nice pay increase and annual bonuses. I also started regularly winning small amounts in lottery tickets. The "abundance" just showed up, and continues to this day.

Sometimes, I can't even give money away without it coming right back to me! Shortly after I finished treatment and was starting to get back to a regular routine, a friend called me with the good news that, after years of unemployment, she was called in for a job interview the next day. She asked if I had a professional outfit she could borrow. Unfortunately, I did not have anything suitable in her size. I had, however, just won $200 on a scratch-off lottery ticket earlier in the day, and I gladly offered it to her. After dropping the winning ticket off at her house, I decided to buy another ticket. It, too, was a $200 winner! The great news is that my friend got the job and had enough of the $200 left to buy an additional work outfit for herself and something special for her son, plus I still had $200 extra for myself! You could attribute this to just plain ol'e dumb luck, or karma rewarding me for my generosity, but I know that all of this happened because of my belief, *I have an abundance of money.*

When facing the biggest fight of your life, and knowing that your behaviors always mirror your thoughts, do you want to unconsciously allow your hurt and scared inner child to make your decisions? Or do you want to intentionally and consciously choose the thoughts and beliefs that will put you on course to get the results you want?

3

CHOOSE YOUR OUTLOOK

Having a positive outlook is one of the most important aspects of overcoming adversity. Whether you focus on the positive aspects of your current situation, or on the positive outcome you expect, you will have a more positive attitude. Conversely, focusing on the negative will not only attract a negative outcome, you will be miserable throughout the experience. I came across a quote a while ago that describes this concept perfectly:

> *"The world is full of cactus, but we don't have to sit on it."[1]*

As I said in the first chapter, I clearly remember the day I was diagnosed with rectal cancer. The doctor said, "I'm sorry, you have cancer." Then he immediately said, "But you are lucky. This is one of the curable cancers. You are not going to die, and when we are finished, you will be cured, not just in remission." I held onto that statement as a lifeline.

I never wavered in my belief that he was right. I even did my own online research which said colon and rectal cancers cause 8.8% of cancer deaths, and the five-year survival rate (the percentage of people who are alive five years after diagnosis) is only 36% for stage III colon and rectal cancer. In spite of this research, my mind, heart, and body were in alignment that I would be cured.

I know that not many doctors will assert so boldly that they will cure you, and very few of the adversities we all face have a guaranteed positive outcome. What do you do when no one gives you a definitive statement to cling to like I had? **You need to look within and find the positivity, self-assurance, and determination necessary to be successful.** If there is any chance of success, focus your attention on a positive outcome. I am not saying that you should live in a dream world. If your goal is to be 5'10," and you are only 5' 3," believing positively that you will grow seven inches just isn't going to work. **Sometimes, a positive attitude simply entails embracing and celebrating the situation you are in, and living each day to its fullest, without worry, fear, or regret.**

I cannot say that I have always had a positive attitude. It could be better described as an accepting attitude: "Whatever is meant to happen, will happen." This *c'est la vie* attitude had allowed me to float along life with ease, albeit sometimes with boredom. My general thoughts had been: *If I am not getting exactly what I want in life, at least what I have is not too bad. If what I want is getting too difficult, maybe it isn't what I really need after all.*

The perfect example of this was my first year of college. My parents couldn't afford to pay for my college, and I didn't want to go into debt to pay for it, so I had applied for several scholarships and grants. I had won an academic scholarship that paid tuition to our local community college for one semester, for which I was extremely grateful. I had a full course-load, plus I was working part-time. I became overwhelmed; there just wasn't enough hours in the day. I ended up dropping one class after a few weeks.

The next semester, I jumped on an opportunity to begin working full-time in order to gain financial independence. When college became overwhelming, I quickly convinced myself that it wasn't my highest priority after all. I first dropped to part-time, then quit altogether. After a little time to mature and to develop the changed perspective that experience brings, I finally got my degree seventeen years later.

In retrospect, I realized that my story of *not good enough* had been at play in dictating my attitude—giving me permission to change my mind about what I wanted early enough to avoid failure. What made me change my perspective was a comment made by the eight-year-old son of a good friend. We were at a barbecue, and his dad asked him what he wanted to do next — toss the football around or play with the Frisbee. He was trying to say either, "I don't care," or "it doesn't matter," but mixed up the two and said, "I don't matter." That was heartbreaking for me, and I wanted to scoop him up and smother him in love, affection, and attention.

I have often felt that I don't matter. I realized three things: that no child should ever feel that they do not matter; that I matter, (regardless of what my inner child might be whispering in my ear); and that I deserve to ask for what I want. That is where the positive attitude comes into play. Once you dare "to want," believing that you will succeed is a must.

Daring to want, but believing that you can't have it will make you miserable. A friend recently posted an old English proverb on Facebook:

"If I were to fall backwards, I would break my nose." [2]

Several people commented, trying to decipher its meaning, but I think it means the writer is so pessimistic that he believes the worst and most improbable consequence will always happen to him. I can't imagine living in such misery.

I have a cousin who survived cervical cancer and

is now in remission, but she lives every day in fear that the cancer will return. For weeks prior to her quarterly blood work and oncology appointments, she is a basket case: she can't eat, she can't sleep, she worries herself sick, and is completely miserable for weeks at a time. She may never have a recurrence, but she is living like she has a death sentence.

On the opposite end of the spectrum, I have a co-worker who survived throat cancer, only to be diagnosed with colon cancer three years later. He did not spend a single day worrying that the cancer might return. He said to me, "Kelly, I **lived.** I spent the last three years enjoying and appreciating life to the fullest. I know I am going to beat it again. But if I don't, it's okay because I have lived a lifetime these past years."

You tell me who has chosen to sit on their cactus! Decide which outlook will make you happiest:

> *"I don't matter. I don't deserve happiness.*
> *I will probably die. Life sucks."*

> *...or...*

> *"I matter. I deserve to be happy. I will be*
> *healed. Life is precious."*

Choose. It is that simple.

4

STRENGTHEN YOURSELF: PREPARE FOR BATTLE

It is important to take care of all aspects of your being. You should be mentally, emotionally, spiritually, and physically ready to battle for what you want. For that matter, why wait? Strengthen yourself now rather than wait for a battle to show up.

Mental: It seems that, from the earliest age, I have always wanted to know as much as I can about everything. "Knowing" helped give me a sense of control; if I could understand it and take away the mystery, then the situation wasn't so scary. After diagnosis, I researched every aspect of the disease and treatment, checking every source I could think of. It was just second nature for me to ask questions of every doctor, nurse, aide, and technician I came across during my recovery, and to continue asking until they offered an explanation that made sense to me.

For those of you who have had a colonoscopy, you know that you are given "twilight" drugs — just enough to completely relax you, but not enough for you to be entirely asleep. Apparently, I drifted off to sleep for a minute or two, and when I awoke, I watched the monitor for the rest of the procedure, but I don't clearly recall any of it.

The nurse made the comment afterwards, "You sure were chatty." When I asked her what she meant, she said that, after the first few minutes, I asked questions non-stop: "What's that? What are you doing now? Where is the scope right now? Why does it look like that?" So, even 75% unconscious, I like to know what is going on! Instinctively, I recognized the importance of being mentally prepared for anything and everything that might occur.

Emotional: I used two tools to be prepared emotionally. **First, I kept a "cancer journal."** I would start by documenting the facts of what happened that day, then I would pour out the emotions I felt relative to those facts. I used this as a way to sort out my feelings, exploring my triggers and constructing mechanisms, such as humor, to turn them around.

For example, midway through my six weeks of chemo and radiation, I was prone to bouts of uncontrollable diarrhea. I had several accidents, generally at home, but once in public. The public incident occurred at a restaurant during lunch with a work colleague who was visiting from out of town. Although the colleague responded with aplomb, I was terribly humiliated. I was an emotional mess for the rest of the day. That evening, I stuffed my emotions down long enough to document what happened and why, reminding myself it was a natural and expected side effect of treatment, and then I let the emotions out! I poured my heart out onto paper. During the writing, a funny little thought hit me, connecting the toxicity of the chemo drugs to body waste, and I started writing about needing a hazmat suit and a special license to dispose of the toxic waste. For some reason, that tickled my funny bone in just the right way, and the next time an accident happened, I was able to giggle my way through cleaning the bathroom floor.

An added benefit of keeping a journal is the power the written word has on your subconscious. Taking the time to write down your new, productive thoughts and the coping mechanisms you have constructed—rather than simply thinking them— makes a more lasting impression on the emotional centers in your brain.

The second tool I used to remain strong emotionally was to disassociate myself from the disease. I never wrote, spoke, or even thought, the phrase "my cancer." Whenever a fellow patient would talk about his (or her) cancer, I would cringe.

It just seems that if you claim it as "yours," it becomes a part of you forever.

Spiritual: Regardless of your spiritual beliefs, or religious affiliations, it is helpful to have faith in a Higher Power. I am Christian, but I have never been actively involved with any church, nor have I studied the Bible. If you practice other religions, or no religion at all, please do not feel excluded by my beliefs. Being able to turn to a Higher Power through prayer for comfort and guidance, establishing a regimen of meditation to find clarity, or practicing some form of reverent ritual to stay centered, will be extremely helpful. I grew, spiritually, by leaps and bounds throughout my ordeal. My faith in God's ability to heal me carried me through.

I am not someone who can get my mind around faith healing, or believing that I would just one day wake up with fully restored good health. I suppose that maybe it is possible, but only for those who believe—beyond a shadow of a doubt—it is possible. Of course, since I had my doubts, I concluded it wasn't possible for me. However, I had a clear vision that God was working through the hands of the doctors, nurses, pharmacists, aides, technicians, and other caregivers; He would heal me through them. This I believed with my whole being, and **I never once wavered in my belief that God would heal me.**

I must admit that, for a short time before

treatment started, fear of the side effects of treatment overwhelmed me. A few words spoken by the daughter of a close friend helped me to get back on track. I was telling her about my faith and that God would heal me through the hands of the medical staff, but that I was fearful of treatment— that I would be ill and in pain all the time and that I just wouldn't be able to cope.

Her response was, "What makes you think that God wants you to be sick and in pain? He doesn't want you to be broken down, torn up, and miserable. Remember that Jesus died so you don't have to experience all that. When you have faith that He will carry you through, He will." This really caught me off-guard because, although my upbringing in the church taught that Jesus died for our sins so we would not suffer after death, I never made the connection that Jesus suffered so that we wouldn't need to suffer in life. Those few simple words impacted me so profoundly that I did not fear treatment after that, and when things got rough, those words carried me through.

I developed a keen sense of gratitude and appreciation. I believe that if you appreciate all that you have, God will keep sending good things your way. If you are not grateful for what you have, what makes you think you would be grateful for anything else?

Every night during my ordeal, I prayed a

gratitude prayer. I was thankful that I got cancer while I was still young and healthy, allowing me to handle the treatment much better than an older person could. I was thankful for my friends and family who continually demonstrated an outpouring of support, especially my step-mother, who is a retired nurse and cared for me so well as I recovered from surgery. She generously and graciously filled so many roles: nurse, housekeeper, cook, caregiver for my father and, most importantly, supportive and loving mother to fill the gap left by my own mother's absence. I was also grateful for my job that allowed me the freedom of a flexible work schedule, a steady paycheck, and good insurance coverage. Every day, I found something new to be grateful for.

Physical: Regardless of what type of adversity you are attempting to overcome, being physically strong will be a tremendous help. This includes good nutrition and plenty of exercise, plus getting adequate rest. I must admit that this is information I ignored, so I need to position this one as: "Do as I say, not as I do!"

I learned much about nutrition and exercise for cancer patients during my information gathering. In a nutshell, cancer cells thrive on glucose, so eating too many sweets and simple carbohydrates presents cancer with a feast. The cancer-killing cells produced by your own immune system thrive on oxygen, so doing some form of cardio exercise, or even deep-breathing exercise, makes them stronger. A combination of overindulging in sweets and not exercising allows cancer cells to set up a comfortable house for which your immune system is not strong enough to evict them. In spite of this knowledge, I gave myself every excuse possible to eat sugary snacks and be sedentary. In this one area, I became a "victim" to the cancer.

Because I did not act on the information I found regarding nutrition and exercise, I struggled physically, at several points during treatment. The cancer was Stage III. This means the tumor was not just in the inner lining of the rectum, but also in the fatty tissue and musculature of the rectum—and had spread to the lymph nodes. As a result, the surgery was much more invasive than Stage I or Stage II cancer would have required, and my treatment consumed just over one year.

It started with six weeks of chemo and radiation, followed by one week of recovery. This was followed immediately with a minor surgery that required two weeks of recovery, then seven weeks of "normal life."

After that, I had my big surgery with ten weeks of recovery; and then, lastly, six months of chemo. Had I only been at Stage II, I could have avoided the final six months of chemo. The initial six weeks of chemo and radiation went well, for the most part. The final week was very difficult, as I will explain in a later chapter, but I did not expect the week after the last treatment to be so awful.

My final treatment was on a Tuesday and, for a full week, I barely left my bed. If I made it out of bed at all, you would likely have found me on the sofa. I was just miserable from the cumulative effects of chemo and radiation. Then one week later, on Wednesday, as soon as I woke up in the morning, it occurred to me that I finally felt well! No pain, no muscle fatigue, and lots of energy. But then that moment of euphoria was immediately followed by realization that I was scheduled for surgery on Friday, just two days away. I know that if I had limited my sugar intake and gotten some form of exercise during the six weeks of chemo and radiation, that final week of treatment, and the next eight days, would not have been quite so difficult.

The same goes for the time between surgeries. After the two weeks of recovery following the first surgery, I went back to work for seven weeks while waiting for the major surgery. I could have had much more energy and stamina than I did during those nine weeks if I had been eating properly and getting plenty of exercise. And I must say that, during the final six months of chemo, I actually gained over thirty pounds, so it is evident that I did not employ any nutritional common sense.

In retrospect, I cannot believe I let myself get away with that behavior! The sad thing is that I got all of my friends and family to buy into my excuses, so no one tried very hard to get me to do the right thing. I am not blaming anyone else for my poor choices because I know that if my intention had been to eat nutritious foods and to exercise, they would have supported my determination to do just that. I am simply commenting on how easy it is for loved ones to accept destructive behavior in the name of sympathy and support, leaving the responsibility for healthy choices wholly up to you.

5

HAVE YOUR FEELINGS; DON'T LET THEM HAVE YOU

One of my favorite quotes is from an unlikely source, LL Cool J. He said,

> *"When adversity strikes, that's when you have to be the most calm.*
> *Take a step back, stay strong, stay grounded, and press on."* [1]

It is okay to feel anger, fear, and self-pity; don't pretend to be happy about your circumstances if you are not. **Give yourself permission to feel your feelings, even the ones that seem dark and scary, but do so intentionally.** Don't let the darkness take you over.

This is a lesson that I learned the hard way many years ago. During my mid-30s, I sunk into a depression. What precipitated it was three "betrayals" that happened nearly simultaneously and completely knocked me off my feet: a boyfriend broke up with me, a friend stole money from me, and my manager didn't seem to appreciate my work any longer. I became mired in a repeating loop of *how could you* and *I don't deserve this*. I really should have sought professional help because I was stuck in this very dark place for nearly six months. Thoughts of suicide were my every day companions. The only joy I had was fantasies of how badly my three betrayers would feel when they learned of my death.

I tried to hide the depression from certain people, like my parents and co-workers, but let my misery show to others. On a typical work day, I would force myself to go into the office and put on a happy face, completely hiding everything I was feeling. The minute I got into my car to drive home from work, however, I would start crying— irrationally bemoaning the fact that no one at work cared enough about me to see through the mask and realize that something was wrong.

Once home, I would either binge-eat sugary foods, (a complete package of Oreo Double-Stuffs was my "drug" of choice) or I would go straight to bed and cry myself to sleep. Both of these were mechanisms I had constructed to avoid my painful thoughts and feelings, and to fill the void created by loneliness and isolation.

On weekends, I got out of bed only to use the

bathroom and to get more junk food. I didn't cook a single meal or clean my house for weeks at a time, and I left the house only for work or to get food.

Most telephone conversations with friends and family inevitably turned to my woe-is-me story. I would repeatedly express my anger and hurt over the betrayals, then turn it into *"what's wrong with me"* hysteria. But I refused to listen to any advice or accept any guidance; in fact, I barely heard it.

But then, after nearly six months of this, a friend found the courage to confront me. She said something to the effect of, "Kelly, get over it already. You are bringing everyone down. No one wants to talk to you anymore because you are such a downer. Either do something to change your situation, or shut up about it." Her tough love was what finally brought me back to awareness.

I believe that this friend helped me to see that, all along, there had been many hands extended into my emotional pit as a lifeline; Divine Grace gave me the strength to finally grab hold and pull myself out.

The first step was to forgive my "betrayers," as I thought of them. I forgave them for treating me so badly. It wasn't long, however, before I realized how shallow and self-righteous this felt. I could finally see how I had created everything that had happened.

For weeks before the breakup, I had become

erratic, jealous, and paranoid around my boyfriend. Keep in mind that this was not a serious relationship; it was just two people who enjoyed spending time together. We were not exclusive and there was no talk of going beyond casual dating. I could finally see how my behavior took the fun out of the relationship, setting it up to end badly.

With the friend who stole money from me, I had been ignoring my intuition and warning signs about her for months. I knew she used people, and I knew she didn't live by the same moral code that I did. Still, I foolishly let her move into my home and was careless about protecting my personal information and money.

With my manager at work, I could finally admit that I hadn't been giving my best effort for months and had not produced any results that deserved appreciation.

The next step was to finally forgive myself. I forgave myself for the actions that precipitated the so-called betrayals. I forgave myself for holding on to the hurt, anger, and bitterness for so long. I forgave myself for spreading misery. And I made a decision at the core of my being to never again let my feelings take complete control like that.

Fast forward to my battle with cancer, I did experience a few instances of extreme emotion but I did not let them take me over. In the early days after diagnosis, and during my treatment regimen, I had moments when the emotions coalesced into a maelstrom of tears. I often found myself bursting into tears while driving home from a doctor's appointment. I would be sobbing so hard I had to pull over to the side of the road until the storm passed, for fear of getting into a car accident. But, by the time I got home, my head was clear and I was able to focus, once again, on the next step. Other times, I intentionally and deliberately shut down my emotions because the immediate situation called for logic, not emotion. I became an expert at compartmentalizing — allowing myself to fully experience moments of joy, hope, faith, and gratitude, but repressing fear, anger, sorrow, and self-pity. In the moment it seemed the right thing to do; in retrospect, I may have suppressed those emotions too often.

Even three years after my cancer battle, they still caught me unaware. Upon learning that a friend from high school was diagnosed with breast cancer, all of those feelings came rushing to the surface. I spent several days in emotional turmoil, reliving my own experience. However, I finally recognized that the suppressed fear and anger had been leading me to make poor choices, which I will discuss in a later chapter. Imagine taking the lid off a container of food that has been hiding in your fridge for months:

the experience is unpleasant, to say the least, but you finally get the putrid food disposed of properly.

Find what works for you; experience your feelings instead of shutting down, but don't let them take you over completely. Instead, **use your emotions as the impetus needed to move you forward on your journey.**

6

REFUSE TO QUIT, GET BACK UP

I think I handled my treatment pretty well, and I never gave up. I came close to quitting one time. As mentioned previously, I initially needed thirty radiation treatments (five days a week for six weeks) with chemo running non-stop via a continuous-infusion pump. By the time I completed the 20th radiation treatment, my skin was burned, I was feeling tired all the time, and I had diarrhea every day. Remember, I had rectal cancer, so the radiation was directed at my bum. Now combine the radiation treatments with a painful tumor, a bad burn, and diarrhea (all concentrated in a single body part) and you can imagine the discomfort—no, that is too mild a description—imagine the pain I was experiencing!

When I showed up for the 28th treatment, the machine malfunctioned, and I was required to wait nearly an hour. I was ready to walk out and skip treatments twenty-eight, twenty-nine, and thirty. I was in the waiting room, in misery, and I decided I just couldn't do it any longer, no matter the consequences, even death. (Yes, it was all quite melodramatic!) I spoke to one of the radiation technicians, telling him that I had to leave and wouldn't be back.

He talked me into staying until he could page my doctor. The radiation oncologist, the kindest and most empathetic person I have ever met, convinced me that I was strong enough to withstand the final three treatments. I don't remember exactly what he said that kept me going; I think I just needed someone to hold my hand and tell me I was strong enough to finish.

Knowing he had faith in me gave me the courage I needed to rejoin the fight.

When the going gets tough, (and it will) and we want to quit, we need to find something, anything, either within or outside of ourselves, to keep us motivated. Quitting is not an option when the stakes are so high.

I mentioned before that my mother died from cancer. She is a great example of what happens when you do give up. She bravely fought cancer for more than ten years. When she was first diagnosed with vulvar cancer (a type of cancer that starts out resembling skin cancer in the female genital area), her oncologist told her that the cancer would not kill her; she would die from "old age" first. (She was in her early fifties at the time.) He recommended surgery because the cancer, if not treated, would eventually become painful. She had her first surgery to remove all damaged tissue, recovered quickly, and lived cancer-free for nearly ten years.

Then the cancer came back. This time her new doctor told her it would advance both outward (covering more surface area of the skin) and inward (into the fatty tissue and ultimately into internal organs). She had another, more invasive, surgery to remove more damaged tissue as well as scar tissue that had resulted from the first surgery. This recovery was not easy; she struggled for nearly six months with wound healing, only to learn that the cancer had already reappeared.

I accompanied her to an oncology appointment where the doctor told her that the cancer was now very aggressive, and there was nothing further that could be done. Another surgery was out of the question, and chemotherapy and radiation treatments had not been proven to have a significant impact in stopping this type of cancer. His prognosis for her differed from what she was told ten years earlier: he predicted she had only six months left to live.

My mother lived in misery for the next six months. She experienced no hope and only fleeting moments of happiness; she became a shell of her former self while waiting to die. Almost six months to the day, my mother lost her battle and passed away. I truly believe that she had convinced herself, at the very core of her being, that she was only going to live for six months, and thus caused it to be true. I am not saying in the literal sense that her death resulted from giving up; her death was caused by incurable cancer. I do, however, believe that she figuratively died on the day she received the six-month prognosis. As soon as she gave up hope that she could beat the disease, she ceased to live fully. I also think that she died on that specific day because she believed she was supposed to.

During those six months, and for a while after her death, I was angry with her for not fighting hard enough and for quitting the battle. Now, with the perspective of twelve years and some life-changing experiences of my own, I am no longer angry with her, and I do not judge her. She made the decision, whether consciously or unconsciously, that she no longer wanted to live with cancer, and that decision played itself out. As much as I miss her, and would give nearly anything to have her back, I think she accepted the consequences of "quitting" with a sense of relief.

7

HONOR RELATIONSHIPS

Spend time with optimistic and successful people. You tend to rise or sink to the energy level of those you surround yourself with. If the adversity you are facing is cancer, it is so important to speak with people who are nearing the end of their treatment cycle. Ask about their stories, find out how they dealt with the disease and the side-effects of treatment as well as life lessons they may have learned. If you are facing some other challenge, speak with people who have overcome similar issues to help keep yourself motivated and to get fresh ideas you may not have thought of on your own. And tell your story to anyone who asks. You may be just the inspiration they need.

My very dear friend, Rita, with whom I will talk about in more detail shortly, was diagnosed with breast cancer just as my treatment was successfully ending. She brings tears to my eyes every time she says this, but she gives me credit for her belief that she would win her battle. She says that my practical approach to beating cancer and my optimistic attitude helped her to face every day with the very same look-forward attitude. I am happy to report that all tests and scans show that Rita has won her battle too!

Don't isolate yourself. Sometimes we feel like hiding from the world when things are not going our way. For me, that old story from my childhood about being *not good enough* made me want to stay at home, alone, when I wasn't feeling my best. The irrational thought was that if they (whoever "they" are) couldn't see me when I was ill, or tired, or grumpy, they would never have an opportunity to judge me. The comfortable and protective mask I had adopted over the years to hide *not good enough* was to be invisible. Most often I would be physically invisible by staying away from people, but I would also be emotionally invisible by not connecting with anyone in the room. I was the classic example of a wallflower. When I was diagnosed with cancer, it was my natural reflex to isolate myself until I felt better — both emotionally and physically. During treatment, I had to make intentional choices to stay out of that mindset. It was difficult, but I accepted nearly every invitation when I felt well enough to do so; if I didn't feel well enough to leave the house, I instead invited them to visit me. In many cases, I kept the visit short, but sharing even 15-20 minutes with a good friend kept my spirits up and helped me to stay focused. Staying connected with the world around me, and being involved in the lives of others, helped me to keep my journey in perspective.

Know who you can count on for emotional and physical support, and lean on them. At the same time, determine (early on) who is NOT part of your support network, so that you do not end up resenting them when they do not meet your high expectations. I have some very close friends who I thought would stick to me like glue. But in reality, they seemed to fall off the face of the earth after I told them of my diagnosis. Perhaps they had painful experiences with the disease, or loss in the past, and simply were not prepared emotionally to face it again. Perhaps their own lives had too many issues and challenges that rightfully had to take priority. Regardless of the reasons, I neither judged nor resented them, and my relationship with each remains on solid ground. I had more than enough people form a support network for me, as I will talk about shortly.

After diagnosis, I had to undergo a major shift in how I looked at "help." I have always been a very independent person. I never asked anyone for help or favors. And if anyone offered to help me with something, I generally refused. To me, offers of help were a sure indication that the person offering help had deemed me "not good enough" to handle it on my own. I knew I had to change this belief immediately, and I learned the lesson in a very remarkable way.

As mentioned previously, when I was diagnosed, I was living in London, England. To show just how independent and averse to help I was at the time, for several days I toyed with the idea of staying in London to continue working throughout treatment. (Remember, I had no family with me in London, and my only friends were work colleagues who would be focused 100% on a successful Olympics. So I would have had no one to help me physically, or provide emotional support during treatment.) The only thing that brought me to my senses was realizing that my health would get worse before it would get better, and I was already struggling to find enough energy to simply function, let alone work the crazy hours the job demanded.

I finally decided that I wanted to come home to Michigan where I would have the support of friends and family. There was one snag, however: I did not have a place to live in Michigan. I knew that I would be staying with my dad and step-mother while recovering from surgery. I didn't want to go through the exercise of finding an apartment that would sit empty for those several months after surgery—but I also didn't want to live with my parents throughout the entire process.

That was when I learned how much my friends care about me. One friend, Brenda, had a condo which had been empty for several years because she moved out of state for her job and had been unable to sell it during the recession. Brenda invited me to live in her condo for as long as I needed. A group of friends, a women's support group I have belonged to for years, got the condo move-in ready for me. It had been used solely for storage for more than three years and really needed a lot of work.

Unbeknownst to me, they cleaned, and cleaned, and cleaned some more to make it ready for me. They donated furniture and household goods for my use. (All of my belongings were still in storage in New York where I had been living before moving to England.) Their labors touched my heart so deeply; I will never be able to fully express my gratitude for them. It was clear that their efforts were not because they thought I couldn't handle things on my own; instead, it was the only way they could think of to express their love for me.

Another example of my support system involves my friend, Rita. When I no longer felt well enough to drive, she became my "chemo companion." She drove me to treatment on many occasions, putting her life on hold so she could keep me company during the very long days at the infusion center. We had some very enjoyable conversations; she told me so many stories and steered the conversation in such interesting directions (national and local politics, religion, relationships, education, among other things) that I became a much more worldly person as a result. The "old me," the one who never accepted help from anyone, would have felt like an imposition on her. I would have been ashamed of needing help, would have been emotionally closed down, and thus would have prevented such enjoyable experiences from occurring.

A final story about my support network involves my older sister, Crystal. She drove me to treatment and to doctors' appointments several times. As a child, I was her biggest fan. I so admired her. She was pretty, she was athletic, and she was popular— all of which I was not. I followed her around so much that I know I annoyed her to no end.

As we became adults, we drifted apart. She moved out of state, got married and started a family, while I pursued my career. We truly became strangers. I am ashamed to say that, over the years, I developed several negative assumptions about her... that she was selfish and self-absorbed, shallow, and one-dimensional. When she volunteered for the first time to take me to an appointment, I was shocked. But I gratefully accepted, and was so very happy to get to know her all over again. I had let go of the hero worship that I had as a child, along with the harsh judgment I had as an adult. We had some really great conversations where she proved to me how smart and multi-dimensional she really is. I even learned that she admired many of my traits and accomplishments which I never would have suspected. I can't help but be grateful for this experience that allowed me to connect with my sister as a peer.

I am telling all of these stories to illustrate how important a support network is. There are so many others I am not naming, so many things that were done for me, big and small, but there simply isn't room here to list them all. **I used my network to vent, to bask in the love they so freely offered, and to help keep me focused on the big picture.** I will be eternally grateful to each and every one of them. This experience has helped me to learn that people love to help if given the opportunity; it is a practical way for people to demonstrate how they feel. It is actually a gift to them to allow them to be there for you however that manifests. Give the gift!

8

BE OPEN TO PLAN B

Sometimes, things just don't work out the way you envisioned them. My vision for myself was to be cancer-free and healthy, exactly as I was before being diagnosed. Unfortunately, I learned shortly after diagnosis that, due to the location of the tumor, I would need a colostomy. For those who don't know, a colostomy is the re-routing of the colon to an artificially created opening in your abdomen called a stoma (colon + stoma = colostomy). A person with a colostomy needs to keep a bag taped to their abdomen, over the stoma, for the collection of body waste. It took a while for me to accept that I would need a colostomy. (I mean, *really*, who *wants* to live with a "poop bag" taped to their belly?) But, ultimately, I decided that I would rather live with a colostomy than die without one.

My radiation oncologist made a comment one

day that, although the radiation was doing a great job at shrinking the tumor (thus improving the odds of a successful surgery), he didn't think there was any way to avoid the colostomy.

When I told him that I had already come to terms with that, and mentioned the desire to live—even if it meant living with a colostomy—he was impressed. He asked if I would be willing to speak with another patient of his. This patient was close to my age and was also facing the need for a colostomy, but was refusing. He would rather die than live with a colostomy.

Of course, I agreed to speak with him. But, unfortunately, he was not willing to do even that. I sincerely hope that, eventually, he came around to the realization that he did want to live, even with a colostomy, and I pray that he is now fully recovered and as happy as I am with Plan B.

Another example of having a Plan B involves my younger sister, Renee. Renee has always wanted to be a mother. She has so much love to give, and she longed for a child to nurture. She married a wonderful man several years ago, and they had been trying to get pregnant ever since. When it didn't happen within a reasonable time, they saw a fertility specialist, and ended up trying artificial insemination as Plan B. After several attempts this, too, failed to result in pregnancy.

Because the desire to be parents was so strong,

they went on to consider Plan C, adoption. I am happy to report that Plan C has been a huge success. Almost five years ago, they accepted a two-year-old foster child into their family, and the adoption is now finalized. My niece is truly a blessing to the entire family. She is open and loving to all; she simply brings joy to everyone she meets. My sister and brother-in-law have since accepted additional foster children into their home, all of whom have been adopted. Renee's Plan C has resulted in being the proud mother of four children!

Sometimes, as described in both examples above, there is simply no alternative than to accept a Plan B (or C). But don't fall into the trap of giving up on Plan A too easily. Be flexible so you can flow around any obstacle that appears instead of getting stuck on it.

Say, for example, your dream is to write a book. You have a general idea of the message you want your book to convey, but the words just aren't coming. Or maybe life gets too hectic, and you find you no longer have the time to invest in writing. Do you give up by saying, "I guess the book just wasn't meant to be?" Do you move to Plan B, which may be writing blogs, articles, or short stories in order to get and keep the creative juices flowing? Or, do you recommit to your passion and move heaven and earth to make the book happen? The answer will be different for each person, because the "truth" of each person's Plan A is different.

What I mean by your "truth" is what you hope to get from it. Only when you are clear on what you hope to get from Plan A can you decide if Plan B still allows you to achieve those results. In the example of writing a book, is your goal merely to write a book? To become famous or rich? Or is it to share a very important message? Understanding the fundamental goal of Plan A will help you to know if Plan B is an acceptable alternative.

To continue with the example of me needing a colostomy, Plan B was easy because it satisfied my underlying needs from Plan A which was to be cancer-free and healthy.

9

BELIEVE IN YOURSELF

Believing in your ability to succeed, no matter what, is critical to overcoming adversity. Rita, about whom I talk so frequently, recently asked me, "What do you know now that you didn't know before?"

My immediate response was, "I know that everything will be okay." But then, before the words were even fully formed, I had to retract them. I had always known that everything will be okay. From the moment I was diagnosed, I knew that everything would be okay. I ultimately changed my answer to Rita's question to, "When I consciously live the belief, *I am able,* there is nothing that I cannot accomplish."

We have all heard the phrase "self-fulfilling prophecy." This means that your beliefs drive your actions and your actions create your life. This happens whether you are on autopilot, letting unknown or hidden beliefs take the wheel, or whether you consciously choose empowering beliefs.

If you believe you will fail, you will unwittingly take actions that will ensure failure. If you believe you are healthy, you will behave like a healthy person, making healthy choices, and thus be healthy. **If you believe that you are able, you will act in an able and capable manner, and you will see success.** This is why so many personal growth and self-help books promote the use of affirmations and positive self-talk.

In all aspects of my life, ever since that episode of depression I discussed in an earlier chapter, I know that everything will be okay. Whenever I encounter (or unintentionally create) a challenge, I know that it will be okay. Whether it is a broken heart (or a bruised ego disguised as a broken heart), a career set-back, a financial crisis, or some other obstacle, after a millisecond of wallowing in that pesky story of *I'm not good enough*, the new belief, *everything will be okay* settles in. As I mentioned previously, with conscious (and sometimes even unconscious) effort, I have been able to turn my bottom-line, destructive self-story of *I'm not good enough* into my highest vision of my highest self, *I am able*.

I am so proud of my sister, Mary, who has finally come around to believing in herself. Mary lost her fiancé to a heart attack a few years ago. Mary is a person who, until this loss, has always been in a relationship. From her first marriage at age eighteen, to her second marriage with a man she met just weeks after her divorce was finalized, to her year-long relationship with her now-deceased fiancé, she has never been alone. She can now clearly see that her beliefs about her own self-worth caused her to jump into relationships, contributed to the ultimate demise of the relationships, and kept her in the relationships well past their expiration dates.

Mary found her own strength about seven months after Mike's passing. She had been living by herself during those seven months, and was struggling with both loneliness and the realities of being alone. It all became too much when she had a flat tire on her way home from work around 10:00 p.m. one night. It was abundantly clear that she had no one to take care of her. After a few moments of grieving for Mike, she pulled herself together and took care of the problem. She finally realized that she can count on herself to not just cope with, but to completely resolve, any challenge that comes her way. It was very empowering for her, for the first time ever, to fully believe in herself.

Folks, this is so important: **find your story that supports your highest self, the one that will trump every other story you have ever told yourself, so that you will believe you can create that which you say you want.**

10

HONOR YOURSELF AND CELEBRATE YOUR SUCCESSES

Acknowledging how successful you have been is critical. Now is not the time for humility or false modesty. **Celebrate, honor, and respect where you have come from, and where you currently are on your journey.** If you think that you are simply not a successful person, that your journey has not been noteworthy, or that your successes are not worth celebrating, think again!

I celebrated and shared many milestones, even small ones, via Facebook. I posted when I was one-quarter, then half-way, then three-quarters, and finally completely through chemo and radiation; I posted when I got out of the hospital after surgery; I even posted when I was able to walk all the way to the end of the driveway and back for the first time.

I previously mentioned having once lost seventy pounds. At the beginning of my weight loss journey,

I took measurements of every part of my body. Every time I started to get discouraged, or hit a plateau, I reminded myself of my progress by holding the tape measure out to my old measurements and measuring the empty space that resulted from my weight loss. Seeing proof positive of my success was so rewarding, and helped me to recommit to my goal. Every time you celebrate a success, you renew your momentum. This is not being boastful, or vain. When you shout, either figuratively or literally, *"I am successful!"* the Universe hears you and sends more success your way.

As I was nearing the end of treatment, I learned that my nephew, his wife, and his in-laws were participating in a Relay for Life sponsored by the American Cancer Society. The event was held on an off-chemo weekend (I had treatment alternating Fridays during that time), so I decided to attend. My intentions were to simply show up and thank them for their fundraising efforts, then make a quick departure so I could take advantage of feeling well by doing something "fun." But, then, things changed. As I was signing in and receiving my survivor's T-shirt, I was asked how long I have been a survivor. My response was "I'm not one yet – I am going to be a survivor, but I still have three months of treatment to go."

The volunteer said, "Oh, no... **every day you live after diagnosis makes you a survivor.**" The emotion welled up in me as I finally started to view myself as a "cancer survivor" rather than a "cancer patient," and I thought back on all of the days I had survived.

A short while later they held the "Survivor's Lap" of the Relay, where survivors and their caregivers were asked to walk the course. Supporters and other Relay participants lined the course and cheered the walkers. This was one of the most awe-inspiring moments of my life: having both loved ones and total strangers cheer me on, honoring me and celebrating all that I had accomplished, and reminding me that the finish line was so very close. This entire experience, plus the slogan for that year, "Celebrate, Remember, Fight Back," caused me to know, deep inside, that I was, and always will be, a survivor. Tears of joy were pouring down my cheeks which were getting sore from smiling so broadly. I was an emotional mess for the rest of the day, but a good mess!

11

LEARN FROM YOUR EXPERIENCE; USE YOUR EXPERIENCE TO HELP OTHERS

After overcoming adversity, some people find that they are changed forever. Something that Walt Disney said rings true:

"All the adversity I've had in my life, all my troubles and obstacles have strengthened me... you may not realize it when it happens, but a kick in the teeth may be the best thing in the world for you."[1]

I got cancer at the time in my life that I was most prepared to battle it. Had I not already experienced and learned from depression, and had I not already done the personal-growth work that helped me understand and change damaging beliefs, my battle with cancer might not have gone so well. The timing was also perfect as it relates to Rita. She was diagnosed with breast cancer just a few months before I finished my treatment, thus allowing me to be healthy enough to reciprocate the support she had given me during my most difficult phase. My successful battle with the disease not only gave Rita the courage and optimism to fight her battle, it gave her first-hand insight into what to expect for herself, and gave her someone supportive who fully understood what she was going through every step of the way. Like my dad, but with a very different meaning and with love in her heart, Rita also says, "Kelly, I'm glad you got cancer."

I would never wish cancer on anyone, nor would I invite it back into my life. However, I would not be the person I am today had I not had cancer. I am stronger mentally, emotionally, and spiritually. I am more willing to offer my opinion because, now, I know that I have valuable insights to offer. I am more compassionate, more empathetic, and more intuitive. I am smarter, and although I am not ready to apply to medical school, I know more about cellular biology and anatomy than any lay person has a right to. I also understand myself and my motivations better than I ever did before. And finally, **I am more willing to take a risk — to pursue my dreams now, rather than wait for "someday."**

I am not saying I am perfect. In fact, I am far from it. For example, I believe my experiences should have made me more tolerant of others who are not feeling well. However, in the last years of his life, when my dad allowed his blood sugar to drop too low, he would get mean. If he snapped or shouted at me, or anyone else in the vicinity, I would snap right back. Then he would start crying, and I would feel like a monster. I know that low blood sugar caused his mood swings, and I should have been more patient; however, I would get frustrated that he didn't monitor his glucose levels closely enough to prevent the radical highs and lows. This was fully within his control, yet he did nothing to manage it.

All I can say is that I continue learning and practicing tolerance and patience, and hopefully, when appropriate, I can help others see what their choices are doing to themselves and help them to seek change.

Even now, I am learning from the very experience of writing this book. As I near the end of my story, I realize how many times I mention my weight, nutrition, and overeating. When I wrote about forgiving myself for so many things as I was coming out of depression, I realized that I have not yet forgiven myself for mistreating my body so badly with binge eating. When I wrote about gaining thirty pounds during the final six months of chemo, I realize that, in the moment, it felt like I deserved to indulge in whatever food I wanted because of all I had been through. When I wrote about the poor choices I made out of suppressed fear and anger, those poor choices related to food.

In retrospect, I realize that I was, once again, dangerously mistreating my body. Weight has always been a struggle for me. As an adult, my weight has fluctuated between 160 and 245 pounds. I am currently at 215 pounds and am striving to get below 200 because I feel so much healthier under that weight. I realize that the only way I can do this is to stop using food as reward or as punishment, and to mask unpleasant emotions.

When I was at my fittest, I chose to eat only foods that supported my health; food filled no other purpose than to provide nutrition. I came to love the taste of fresh, whole foods, and I craved the euphoria and sense of power that came with exercise.

The experience of writing a book about my battle with cancer has allowed me to compassionately come to terms with my emotional connection with food. I finally forgave myself for years of mistreating my body which contributed to the development of cancer in the first place. And I commit, once again, to make healthy food choices.

It also gives me an opportunity to beta test all the concepts I am writing about; I will see if following my own advice will result in successfully overcoming obesity. By the time I finish writing, I intend to have reached my goal of weighing less than 200 pounds, and being well on my way to developing healthy habits that will last a lifetime.

As you learn from and share your experiences, I encourage you to give back in some fashion before, during, or after your successful battle with whatever adversity you are facing. For example, if your challenge is that you have lost your job, then encourage and support others who have also lost their job, and pass along any opportunities you learn about to others. If you have lost a loved one, find or start a support group for dealing with similar tragedies. If you battled cancer, contribute time or money to a charitable organization that promotes cancer prevention, funds research toward a cure, or provides financial assistance to cancer patients. There are so many ways you can use your experiences to have a meaningful impact on others. Your generosity and willingness to help others will come back to you in so many tangible and intangible ways.

I tell my story to anyone who will listen. I have given the Survivor's speech at a few American Cancer Society Relays for Life, even though **my story really isn't about beating cancer, it is about finding the right combination of attitude, faith, and strength to beat any adversity.**

I would feel so honored if even one person can learn from my experiences—to help them face cancer, end depression, mend relationships, or find their own self-worth. If sharing my experience helps others to overcome whatever adversity they are facing, then my mission will be complete.

12

CONCLUSION

Cancer sucks! It changes the lives of everyone it touches, not just those who are stricken with the disease, but caregivers and loved ones as well. It is no longer the distant and impersonal killer that I hear statistics about; it is a real-life, personal adversary. I have too many friends and family members battling the disease right now, and I have lost too many loved ones to it. I will strike back at this enemy in every way I can.

If life was like a train on the tracks, I would describe my life before cancer as chugging along across the plains—rather flat and uneventful, but getting to the destination I chose for myself. Then along comes cancer, and I am switched to an alternate track.

This new track is more like a roller coaster, with sharp curves, steep climbs, dramatic drops, corkscrews, and even the big loop where I seem to hang upside down indefinitely. When I reach the apex of the giant climb, I can scream out my fear as I begin the plunge. I can either throw my hands in the air, or I can cling to the safety bar. No one, not even me, will judge my actions. And then, as the ride comes to an end, I am forever changed by the experience. I am no longer satisfied with chugging along the flat and uneventful tracks across the plains. But it is satisfying to know that I can choose which track I want to be on... with a limitless number of options!

My career is not on the same track as it was before cancer, but I love the work I am doing now, and I am gaining experiences I would not have had before. I suspect my future career prospects are even greater than they were prior to cancer. I love, honor, respect, and appreciate the people in my life so much more than I ever did previously, and I am not afraid to express to them how I feel because I was on the receiving end of so much love.

I am following my life's passion: I am finally writing a book. Words have always been my friends, but until my battle with cancer I was never motivated to write because I felt I never had anything important to say.

Now I even have a second book rattling around in my head, and in my heart, because this life experience has been so profound. I no longer feel the need to be "invisible." Rather, I want to connect with and have an impact on others. It has become very clear that I have a choice in every aspect of life including career, finances, relationships, and health (just to name a few).

I wear the scars on my body with pride. The scar on my chest from where the chemo port was; the scar that runs from just below my breasts down to my pubic bone (where skin and muscle tissue was taken for reconstruction); the maze of scars on my bum, and even my colostomy (while not technically a "scar," it is a physical abnormality, so I count it here), **ALL are symbols of strength and survival.**

I recently saw an article about a woman with a colostomy who wore a bikini on the beach while on vacation. The photos made their way to Facebook where they garnered extraordinary comment and feedback. People from around the world have shown their support for her courage in refusing to keep her colostomy hidden in darkness and shame. While I am not quite ready to wear a bikini, I proudly view my colostomy as a way for me to shout, "I am alive!"

So, yes, cancer sucks! So does divorce, loss of a job, death of a loved one, natural disaster, and the list goes on. The good news is that you get to choose how you deal with the situation and how you live in the aftermath of it. Choose well!

ABOUT THE AUTHOR

Kelly Wilton is a cancer survivor who learned some valuable life lessons during her fight with the disease. In her day job, Kelly is a licensed customs broker, working for a global logistics company. Kelly spends most of her time at work translating complex import/export regulations into easy-to-understand, actionable steps for customers and employees. She also enjoys every opportunity to mentor, coach and inspire the next generation of logistics professionals. Kelly's work experience of dealing with complex subject matter, and her desire to use her knowledge to develop others, enabled her to successfully beat cancer and document her experience as a guide for others to follow in her footsteps. Kelly has recently returned to her hometown of Port Huron, Michigan, after spending 3 years in upstate New York and 14 months in London, England. She travels extensively throughout the US for work, and is a respected speaker at logistics industry events.

If you wish to contact Kelly, you may reach her at kwilton234@yahoo.com.

ACKNOWLEDGMENTS

Thank you to...

Ricki and Rita for encouraging me to "dig deeper." And then Ricki reviewed draft, after draft, after draft, offering valuable critique every step of the way.

Sue for critiquing one of the nearly final versions of my book, not letting me get away with sloppy grammar.

My women's group (Ricki, Cindy, Brenda, Kim, Chris, Rita, Dona, Joy) who offered so much support during my cancer battle, then let me ramble on for months about every success and challenge in writing my story.

And finally, my sisters (Chris, Mary, and Renee) for being the living embodiment of many of the concepts included in the book.

NOTES

3. Choose Your Outlook

1. Foley, Will. *Forbes Quotes, Thoughts on the Business of Life*, https://www.forbes.com/quotes/9713/
2. Old English Proverb. https://bit.ly/2W3lTmM

5. Have Your Feelings; Don't Let Them

Have You

1. LL Cool J. BrainyQuote.com.

   https://www.brainyquote.com/quotes/ll_cool_j_417684

11. Learn from Your Experience; Use Your Experience to Help Others

1. Disney, Walt. BrainyQuote.com

   https://www.brainyquote.com/quotes/walt_disney_130929

BOOK SUMMARY

Book Summary

"I'm Glad I got Cancer: A Survivor's Guide to Triumphing Over Adversity" is a guidebook for those facing any difficulty in life, including cancer, divorce, death a loved one, financial hardship, loss of a job, and so on. The story was inspired when the author's father made the bizarre comment, "Kelly, I'm glad you got cancer". It goes on to chronicle Kelly's life experiences that helped her to be well-positioned to face her emotional and physical battle with cancer. It contains specific actions the reader can take to help with their personal challenges, supported by Kelly's personal stories to reinforce the message. While you cannot control the challenges life throws at you, you always have control over your own thoughts, feelings, and actions. Remember, you may be given a cactus, but you aren't forced to sit on it!